Table of Contents

Brain Aneurysm Genetic Testing and Screening Guidelines

1. Introduction to Brain Aneurysms

Today, the primary clinical significance of unruptured cerebral aneurysms lies in the prevention of subarachnoid hemorrhage (SAH) due to its serious consequences. Some patients diagnosed with a cerebral aneurysm in one part of the brain may also have an aneurysm elsewhere. This implies that to detect or rule out any other aneurysms, the person must usually undergo a full brain screening. This CT or MRI scan, often coupled with a cerebral arteriography procedure, brings the cumulative exposure to radiation and the potential risk of damage related to the procedure. In the event of an additional aneurysm, the person will need to weigh the benefits, costs, and potential risks of fixing it. This is why the American Academy of Family Physicians and the Canadian Association for Family Physicians do not recommend selective screening for individuals in the general population when no other clinical signs suggest the presence of the disorder.

A brain aneurysm refers to a weakened, bulging area in the wall of an artery in the brain. They are often described as "berry" aneurysms due to the small, round shape of the bulge. About 6 million people in the United States have an unruptured brain aneurysm. However, like a balloon or a weak spot in a tire, weakness in the wall of an artery can lead to a spontaneous rupture, causing bleeding into the space around the brain or into the brain tissues. If rupture occurs, 40% of patients die, and about 66% of those who survive suffer from some type of permanent neurological deficit. This makes knowledge about cerebral aneurysms critical to health preservation.

1.1. Definition and Types

In the classification devised by Lasjaunias, aneurysms are defined as single-saccular or refractory, i.e. not visualized on angiography, venous plexus aneurysms or arteriovenous phase aneurysms, during which there is pre-thickening of feeders or slow circulation of contrast through the dilatation. More recent advances in the understanding of aneurysm pathogenesis are elucidating genetic, hemodynamic, and endothelial factors as well as inflammatory and matrix-degrading mechanisms. Aneurysms can result from constitutional disorders such as Marfan and Ehlers-Danlos syndromes or polycystic kidneys or are caused by spirochetal infection. They may be caused in association with cerebral arteriovenous malformations or parasitic arterial infections, by local or general vasoconstriction due to eclampsia, selective serotonin reuptake inhibitors, smoking, or lack of fit or may be idiosyncratic. The majority of aneurysms are classified as sporadic, i.e. not resulting from an environmental factor.

A brain aneurysm is a bulge in an artery in the brain. Aneurysms can result from arterial wall thinning and ballooning, exerting pressure on brain tissue and acting as a source of potential hemorrhage. Brain aneurysms are generally described on the basis of their shape, septation, and spatial relationship to branch vessels, and classified as either saccular or fusiform/dissecting. Saccular aneurysms generally emerge from a major cerebral arterial bifurcation, extend laterally, and are attached at their base to one of the branches; they are further characterized by short, wide-necked, regular or broad fundus saccular aneurysms, spindly broad-necked aneurysms, and "giant" aneurysms with a maximum diameter of 20, not 25, mm. Auguin classified aneurysms as thin-walled irregular, dumbbell-shaped, and "mycotic" multilocular and mixed masses.

1.2. Epidemiology and Risk Factors

Age in community-based studies appears to have a bimodal distribution with peaks in the 5th and 8th decades, with a mean age of about 60. Aneurysmal SAH among individuals >65 years is often attributed to underlying systemic mechanisms. Other lifestyle risk factors for local aneurysm disease in the general population include the female sex as well as Caucasian race. In general, women are more likely to develop aneurysms than men, and a larger proportion of postmenopausal women develop aneurysms and aneurysm rupture than premenopausal women. Pre-menopausally, a portion of their female population is "protected" from developing brain aneurysms due to hormone replacement during the menstrual cycle, namely estradiol.

The burden of unruptured and ruptured brain aneurysms in the general population is considerable. A community-based study estimated an overall prevalence of unruptured intracranial aneurysms of 3.3% (95% CI 2.4-4.3), which increased with age. A ruptured brain aneurysm (SAH) is less common than unruptured brain aneurysms, but can lead to devastating long-term disability or death. According to the "Ruptured Aneurysm Global Epidemiology Study" (RAGES), there are approximately 300,000 new cases of SAH globally each year, and an estimated 170,000 (60%) die from the ruptured brain aneurysm. In the U.S., an estimated 30,000 individuals suffer from SAH each year, and worldwide, SAH accounts for 0.9% of all deaths. Most brain aneurysms present as incidental findings, but the risk of rupture has lifelong implications for patients and families. Excessive amounts of cigarette smoking, hypertension, and heavy alcohol consumption are three major risk factors for cortical SAH. Subarachnoid (SAH) and intracerebral (ICH) hemorrhages are ten times more frequent than subdural (SDH) and epidural (EDH) hemorrhages in hemorrhagic genetic vascular disease.

2. Genetics of Brain Aneurysms

Researchers believe that genetic factors alone cannot cause the development and rupture of an intracranial aneurysm, as non-genetic factors also play a role. This is manipulated by testing thousands of functional loci across the genome in subjects with and without aortic aneurysms. Several genes have been associated with the development of intracranial aneurysms, a majority of them also seen in aortic aneurysm patients. However, intracranial aneurysms are not observed in all patients with mutations in a known primary aneurysm gene. Therefore, genetic testing cannot determine if an individual will develop an IA or multiple IAs. Moreover, having an IA is not sufficient to justify genetic testing. Some centers recommend considering testing in those with an IA if individuals have more than one first-degree relative with an ICH or SAH or IA or unruptured aneurysm in individuals under 50 years.

About 2% of the population has an aneurysm, and the lifetime risk for an aneurysmal subarachnoid hemorrhage (aSAH) is estimated at 3%. Though factors like female sex, smoking, high blood pressure, and connective tissue diseases like Ehlers-Danlos or Marfan syndrome all increase an individual's risk for the development of a brain aneurysm, up to 40% of aSAH patients have a family history of the condition, suggesting a genetic basis. On average, first-degree relatives of aSAH patients have a 2-3% risk of harboring an aneurysm, compared to a baseline of 1-2% in the general population. Although clinically used software programs cannot predict aneurysm location, several susceptibility genes and chromosomal loci have been associated with aneurysm formation over the years. These discovery methods continue to evolve as genetic testing and whole genome sequencing (WGS) have become more available as tools for a complete picture of one's risk. As we learn more about the genetics of aneurysms, genetic testing for aneurysms is going to increase in utilization.

2.1. Inheritance Patterns

A few inherited conditions or diseases can include brain aneurysms in affected members of greater than one family generation. They include hereditary hemorrhagic telangiectasia (HHT or Osler-Weber-Rendu syndrome), fibromuscular dysplasia (FMD), and some families with polycystic kidney disease (PCKD). Familial aneurysms fit the model of "multifactorial inheritance," a combination of genetic and possibly environmental factors. Familial brain aneurysms may fit a small part of the "common aneurysm" found in 2% of middle-aged United States families. Copies of useful patient education brochures on some of these conditions are available from the California Department of Public Health (CDPH), Genetic Disease Screening Program.

Familial Aneurysm

Unless brain aneurysms affect many family members and multiple generations, brain aneurysms are not clearly hereditary for most. They can be if they are part of a larger health condition(s). These conditions are diagnosed on additional findings of aneurysms in the aorta (the larger vessel that blood flows through from our heart). In these families, known as vascular connective tissue "syndrome" families, other findings might include easy bruising, thin skin, complications with connective tissues from the head to the toes. There are many potential genetic conditions causing connective tissue findings, it is important to see a genetics professional (geneticist, genetic counselor, or genetic nurse) for possible evaluation. Some inherited conditions are known to cause brain aneurysms in families.

Genetic Factors

Aneurysms form for a variety of reasons such as heart or brain defects from birth (congenital), infections, trauma, fluid in the brain, or abnormal blood flow. Most brain aneurysms are the result of subtle damage to blood vessel walls. Aneurysms may not affect all family members. There are no guidelines to predict if or when a brain aneurysm may develop. Support for Families.

About Brain Aneurysms

2.2. Genes Associated with Brain Aneurysms

A specialized cell in the artery wall called the vascular smooth muscle cell is important in arterial development, as well as in what we commonly refer to as "hardening of the arteries". Changes in an important protein, the vascular smooth muscle cell, from answers to questions about hardening of the arteries has also been observed in cells from brain aneurysms. The Compassionate Allowance program refers to a method of quickly identifying diseases and other medical conditions that invariably qualify under the Listing of Impairments based on minimal objective medical information. This applies not only to the initial determination of disability, but to the individuals who are disabled. The Brain Aneurysm Foundation is hopeful that individuals with suspected familial brain aneurysms (described under Screening Guidelines) will be required to have their brain anatomy imaged and suspect brain aneurysms treated before age 50.

There is likely a genetic component to brain aneurysms. Research is growing on the specific genes that may be linked with the development of brain aneurysms. Only a small percentage of people with the genetic risk will actually have a brain aneurysm, so there are likely to be other genetic and non-genetic factors that are involved. It is not currently recommended to receive brain aneurysm genetic testing except under certain circumstances. Assuming a person does not have a genetic mutation that is linked with IA, brain aneurysms can rupture at any time in life.

3. Role of Genetic Testing

In general, aneurysms need to be fairly large in order to be seen on imaging, unless the imaging has special qualities, like arteries are sought specifically (like certain MRA techniques) or is a higher resolution (like CTA). As anatomical factors like the branching pattern at the location of the aneurysm and the presence of variably sized blood vessels in the brain cause a higher level of variability in which people tend to harbor aneurysms, they are generally not used as general screening tools in a relatively healthy population. Furthermore, large population-based studies suggest that up to 15% of people may harbor brain aneurysms. Currently, before any guideline for imaging based on genetics can be designed, we need further information about how useful this strategy is in improving outcomes and more accurate or individualized risk assessment. It is currently not known if a strategy of standardized or tailored genetic-based screening carries benefits in terms of improving outcomes or quality of life.

There is significant debate about the utility of genetic testing for aneurysms. The largest benefit of genetic testing would be identifying individuals who have an asymptomatic aneurysm simply because they are at increased risk of having one (i.e., without an obvious triggering event). Knowing the genetic underpinning of an individual's aneurysm may also be linked to complications from the aneurysm or guide ultrasonography screening interval. An additional potential benefit of genetic testing is to get a better idea of the familial risk, but this is primarily useful in identifying individuals at increased risk of harboring brain aneurysms.

3.1. Indications for Genetic Testing

Genetic testing should not be undertaken without either imaging to directly demonstrate the presence of aneurysm or moyamoya, or in the presence of international data standards that state which subtype of pathogenic variant is classified and demonstrates a high risk of meeting the diagnostic criteria for this disorder. There is at least one subtype of some syndromes where it is clinically useful to do genetic testing even when the imaging shows no features of that syndrome.

In general, the following patients should be considered for genetic testing: when there is no family history available but an intracranial aneurysm has been documented on imaging for patients less than 60 years of age; in the presence of a first-degree relative with spinal or hypophyseal aneurysms, or where there is a family history of both hemorrhagic and unruptured intracranial aneurysms; for patients with multiple intracranial aneurysms; in the presence of a patient with a young-onset internal carotid artery aneurysm, vascular variants, or a concerning appearance on imaging. In young patients with a normal family history, and a negative twin study, there may be consideration to not proceed with genetic testing. The optimal age is not precisely defined, but an age range of 18–40 years for intracranial aneurysms is often stated, although people with familial and/or heritable syndromes continue to have aneurysms until 55 years of age, so some suggest considering genetic testing after this time range, in such patients.

3.2. Types of Genetic Testing

The most thorough exam looks at a person's entire DNA. The most common tests are known as a "multi-gene panel" or "clinical exome sequencing." A multi-gene panel includes most of the genes that affect or may affect a condition. For people with multiple brain aneurysms, the most appropriate panel includes the most common adult or familial brain aneurysm genes. Many laboratories perform genetic testing. Centers performing testing of people without known brain aneurysm gene in their family include University of Texas Health in San Antonio, Blueprint Genetics, and Fulgent Genetics. Other types of laboratory tests must be ordered by a healthcare professional directly associated with a specific laboratory. Testing to find a mutation (usually in a parent or parents), develop a profile that is then used to test a minor who might have inherited the mutation, is likely the most ethical way to proceed by the family and its healthcare providers. The first step is called a "targeted" test. If the parent's mutation is found, it can be used for predictive testing, or "predictive testing panels" or "DNA banking" in the future. Banked DNA can be used by the person or given to a research lab if the mutation is never found. It usually takes weeks to receive results. This type of test is a "clinical" test in that it uses validated technology and is generally offered to people with an apparent indication that a genetic mutation could be involved in their condition. Generally, a healthcare professional must order testing. Often, genetics counselors help people decide when this, or any, test is appropriate. The many decisions that go into getting genetics testing are often made over two conversations with a genetic counselor, although some people decide to go forward on the first call.

4. Screening Guidelines

Screening is critical to identifying the presence and characteristics of brain AVMs and cerebral aneurysms as early as possible, potentially before symptoms develop. Indications for referral for imaging include clinical signs. Resources for neurologic care with experience in HHT are available to assist healthcare providers in identifying and informing their patients at risk for brain AVM (or PAVM). The risk of initial or recurrent brain AVM bleeding may be sufficient to justify an initial evaluation if presenting symptoms carry a high risk of brain AVM hemorrhage. No fixed age cutoff exists for medical judgment of the necessity for screening, but if data reveal a decreased AVM rupture risk in the elderly, age considerations may be taken into account in these decisions.

The presence, size, and number of brain aneurysms have been shown to be highly variable from family to family and within the same family. The responsibility to identify the individuals at risk and to test only those at risk falls to the multidisciplinary medical team, typically overseen by a neurologist experienced in hereditary hemorrhagic telangiectasia (HHT). Aneurysms can easily be detected by a computed tomography angiography (CTA) or a magnetic resonance angiogram (MRA). It is important to note that the guidelines for screening for aneurysms are specific to each disease. This section provides information for specialists in HHT and in first-degree relatives or offspring. While the guidelines for screening for aneurysms are based on expert opinion rather than scientific studies, the rationale behind them is that smaller aneurysms are less likely to rupture, which is believed to pose the greatest risk in this population, and therefore do not need to be treated.

4.1. Current Screening Recommendations

These guidelines are stratified for smoking habits and hypertension. The U.S. Preventive Services Task Force (draft statement July 2020) does not advise in favor of screening as there are no randomized controlled trials of the effect of screening for aneurysms on the incidence or impact of aneurysmal SAH. Most cerebral aneurysms are asymptomatic and are incidentally found on imaging done for an unrelated reason or after a rupture. Systematic patient screening is a matter of debate. Magnetic resonance imaging (MRI) is the modality of choice for screening of individuals at risk for heritable aneurysm formation, particularly in children and young at-risk adults, to avoid radiation exposure.

Guidelines for deep brain cavernomas and large fluid-attenuated inversion recovery-positive cerebral cavernomas suggest that subjects with a first-degree relative affected with lesions should be screened, with the possibility of inversely tailoring intervals based on the first normal examination if the disease shows reduced penetrance. Genetic counseling can be tailored on the basis of mutation. The Evidence-Based Guidelines for the risk of acquiring aneurysms suggest the screening of subjects having at least two affected first or second-degree relatives. The National Institute for Health and Care Excellence guidelines are based on four expert consensuses (level 4 of evidence) and recommend screening on subjects with at least one affected first-degree relative or at least one second-degree relative with two or more affected. They state that the offspring of parents with an intracranial aneurysm are not at increased risk unless other first-degree relatives are affected.

Current Screening Recommendations

Screening for Brain Aneurysms

4.2. Imaging Modalities for Screening

The utility of CTA often depends on the presence of pre-existing vascular clips in patients who have undergone surgical intervention for coiled aneurysms, given the metal artifact that clips can generate. A CTA is usually sufficient if a patient is screened for genetic predisposition to brain aneurysms. Until a patient is evaluated by MRI/MRA, the possibility of a pre-existing clip in the intracranial circulation may be either fully contraindicated or evaluated based on time after surgery. The interventionalist should be consulted if such a patient is deemed to need MRI/MRA. All first-degree relatives and FDRs should have an aneurysm-screening modality performed before consideration of definitive treatment for the affected proband. This is important due to the theoretical risk of coexisting aneurysm in the caregiver in whom the family is reliant upon for neo-aneurysm treatment, as well as the known risk of sentinel, high grade, potentially catastrophic subarachnoid hemorrhage while the FDR is in the hospital for proband treatment. MRI is particularly important in the patients who are likely to need a stent-assisted therapy for aneurysm if it will be performed at an outside institution, since device selection should be tailored for treating a patient with a computed-aided-stem potentiality of having an intracranial clip. Alternatively, a CTA or MRA may be performed instead of an MRI.

For patients who are at risk for brain aneurysms, several screening tools can be employed. The first screening test is typically a noncontrast head computed tomography (CT) scan, which can be particularly helpful for evaluating patients who present to the emergency department with neurological symptoms. This scan can evaluate for subarachnoid hemorrhage caused by an aneurysm rupture. A cranial magnetic resonance imaging (MRI) or CT angiography (CTA) scan can be performed to visualize the cerebral vasculature.

5. Clinical Implications

Most Ruptured intracranial aneurysm (RIA) has devastating consequences with a death from the initial bleed, regardless of medical treatment, of about 30-50%. 15% of those who survive the initial bleed will have a second bleed within 14 days and even more will have rebleed after that. Patients and families are often looking for definitive, actionable intuitions from gene testing or IS in terms of future IA bleed risk rates. While there are potential treatments available to prevent or treat IAs in the setting of ADPKD-type IA, there are currently no therapies for IS or AD, and only recommendations for 'lifestyle modifications' to reduce natural history rupture risks of unenlarged IAs if discovered on screening/testing. Clinicians can discuss some dangerous uncommon or hypothetical possible treatments as interventions that are discussed below. Clinicians should carefully discuss nonintervention and should discuss and advise against increasing exercise, participating in tackle sports, weightlifting heavyweight resistance training, using vasoconstricting or energy-booster supplements or recreational drugs, or donating a kidney; all of which will increase the risk of catastrophic rupture in those concerned about potential IA risk.

Screening for Unruptured Intracranial Aneurysms

Genetic testing can identify the most common genes associated with IA and can be useful when family history is consistent with an autosomal dominant pattern of inherited risk. For those in whom positive genetic testing results are found for FIA, periodic screening for IAs may be indicated, as well as offered to all first-degree relatives. However, as both FH and DEH are SNHs that can involve multiple different underlying rare gene variants, it is important for patients and clinicians to understand that negative FIA/IA-gene testing does not rule out familial risk for IA.

Genetic Testing

5.1. Management Strategies Based on Genetic Test Results

The ideal approach to the prevention of SAH due to brain aneurysm is, to some extent, a strategy of secondary prevention. The fortunate aspect of the progress in treating HHT has been improved. The main aspect of aneurysm management is the altered strategy for patients who need anti-platelet therapy associated with cerebral embolization. Adult family members of those with tested VUS mutations that suggest increased aneurysm risk are educated about SAH symptoms and signs. Leakage will be formed on the basis of non-prophylactic follow-up of treatment by patient choice if desired, with plans for genome testing again if the aneurysm is detected at the time of leakage. In cases in which it is difficult to decide the contributory risk of the rare genetic variant to aneurysm presence or rupture, the genetic counselor should emphasize that even individuals carrying as yet uncharacterized VUS genetic variants of genes likely to be associated with SAH are not protected from aneurysm formation or rupture.

With the advent of genetic testing for brain aneurysms, a natural response is to adjust and supplement HT guidelines that provide strategies for screening and protecting patients against the threat of aneurysmal SAH. The immediate question that arises is whether adjuvant pharmacologic therapy or intervention should be offered to those who are tested. This section will attempt to build a pragmatic viewpoint of the management of brain aneurysm risk based on genetic test results.

6. Ethical and Legal Considerations

On the other hand, there are ethical and legal considerations when choosing to screen children for adult disease. For treatments where screening is not applicable, it may draw unnecessary attention or fear toward the disease and raise psychological and ethical issues with regard to the parents who decide to exclude the child from this information, even based on national legislation. It is difficult to generalize recommendations for central-state protocols when recent national genomic legislation differs considerably worldwide.

In all hereditary diseases, the main issue remains the right to know or not to know a piece of information, which can strongly impact future health conditions and quality of life. This is the reason for respecting the fundamental right of patients to consent, or not, to genetic testing and the fact that testing should be preceded by genetic counselling. Genetic counseling involves support of the unveiling of the genetic testing results, when requested by the adult patient to know the genetic risks. Current international recommendations aim to ensure that a patient is fully aware of the hourly news about the genetic determinants of the disease in order to make aware and informed consents. Even after the genetic test has been performed, the primary right of a patient is to choose the optimal prevention, treatment, and offensive strategies. The purpose of international guidelines on aneurysm is to stress the importance of screening until adulthood but, unfortunately, the portion of the patient population that starts screening in adult age is still minimal.

6.1. Patient Consent and Genetic Counseling

Waivers for research involving humans frequently have the requirement for informed consent by the subjects to be waived if the subjects are not likely to perceive any adverse consequences from not consenting. This would be particularly relevant in conducting genetic research on samples from deceased cases and the families of deceased cases where there may be little burden on the family by not consenting. Where risk is still present, we would recommend obtaining both written and verbal consent at the time of autopsy by the next of kin for the collection of genetic samples. The issue of consent has often been grounded in the fact that the action is being done on the body or obtaining tissues after death, but for research purposes, an additional factor could be that the data is likely to not directly relate to that individual. The ability to link specific aneurysm features to specific genes, however, may be a strong motivation for obtaining consent for DNA collection.

Patients at greater risk of developing or transmitting an aneurysm (based upon family history) may sometimes wish to have genetic screening in order to determine more specific risk levels. Guidelines have largely converged around the following: 1) making sure that the person knows the limits of what is known and what is not known about genetic causes of aneurysm formation and rupture, and 2) providing genetic counseling for everyone considering brain aneurysm genetic testing. Potential risks are associated with genetic testing or genetic screening.

Consistent with guidance from the International Society of Nurses in Genetics, the "Born with Risk" book recommends that patients who had an aneurysmal bleed strongly consider genetic counseling before proceeding with genetic testing. The guidance additionally is explicit that genetic counselors with special training in neurovascular disorders should provide all brain aneurysm genetic counseling.

Genetic Testing for Brain Aneurysm Risk in Individuals with Family History

1. Introduction to Brain Aneurysms and Genetic Risk Factors

Brain aneurysms are weak bulging spots on the wall of the brain blood vessels. The risk for brain aneurysm formation with rupture increases with age and genetic predisposition is a significant risk factor. Genetic risk factors play a much more significant role in causing brain aneurysms in younger individuals without routine stroke risk profiles such as high blood pressure and smoking history or tend to form in unusual location of brain blood vessels pupillary light reflex. We believe genetic predisposition plays a larger role in brain aneurysm formation in younger individuals and families with multiple affected family members. Brain aneurysm rupture causes brain hemorrhage and affects between 20,000 to 30,000 individuals in the United States each year. Brain aneurysm rupture kills 35-40% of patients, and of the survivors, half are disabled.

Family history of brain aneurysm is a risk factor for brain aneurysm formation, potentially reflecting genetic predisposition in which multiple genetic risk factors inherited among family members contribute. In this study, we aim to identify adults who have at least one family member who has been treated or died from a ruptured brain aneurysm. Our long-term goal is to conduct precision prediction studies in these individuals with increased genetic risk to identify individuals who are much more likely to develop a brain aneurysm based on the inherited genetic risk factors. In particular, our study team aims to identify males who would never be candidates for brain aneurysm section by current guidelines, and identify individuals in the female reproductive age most likely to form a brain aneurysm.

1.1. Definition and Types of Brain Aneurysms

There are two general types of brain aneurysms, saccular and non-saccular, and four subtypes that will be discussed below. The important distinguishing features of the four subtypes are their causes, the location of the aneurysm, and the probability of their occurrence. The medical terms for the aneurysms that happen less often are as follows: fusiform, C-shaped, dissecting, and blister. Each of these conditions will be defined as part of the following discussion.

Brain aneurysms are balloon-like dilations in the wall of a cerebral blood vessel. Most intracranial aneurysms will never rupture. However, any aneurysm has the potential to rupture. When an aneurysm ruptures and bleeds into the space surrounding the brain, this is termed a subarachnoid hemorrhage (SAH). The most dangerous time for the patient is generally the first 24 hours after the bleed. The overall mortality rate for a ruptured intracranial aneurysm is as high as 60%, with reports in the medical literature of between 25-40% of SAH survivors being left with severe (and often lifelong) cognitive deficits and physical disability among survivors.

Family aggregation of brain aneurysms reflects shared risk factors. Shared genetic factors can also influence the initiation and progression of brain aneurysms. Family-based studies have consistently supported a role of highly penetrant genetic variants in brain aneurysm formation. In the reported studies, 7% to 20% of participants self-reported a family history of a brain aneurysm. However, the discovery of genetic variants that underlie familial brain aneurysm formation has been challenging. In contrast, the discovery of genetic variants that increase the risk in a more modest way of developing a brain aneurysm has been relatively successful. This is in part because of a larger population that contributes to sporadic brain aneurysm aggregation. To date, the importance of traditional risk factors (smoking, uncontrolled hypertension) and genomic risk factors explains 20% of the aneurysm heritability, the contribution of genetic factors to the familial aggregation of brain aneurysms. The substantial missing heritability suggests that a large proportion of aneurysm heritability could be explained by both rare anatomical variants and rare and common variants not yet discovered.

Brain (cerebral) aneurysms are weak spots in brain arteries caused by thin walls. They can rupture, leading to devastating outcomes. Only a small fraction of the population has aneurysms, and about two-thirds of the aneurysms diagnosed in people living in the United States are in women. Individuals with multiple relatives who have had brain aneurysms have a substantially higher risk of having a brain aneurysm. However, the disease has low penetrance. Low penetrance means that some individuals with mutations that confer higher vulnerability to aneurysm formation do not get aneurysms; this may be due to additional genetic and environmental factors. While environmental factors are likely to underlie sex and age differences in aneurysm prevalence, genetic factors, including common variants, may also play a role.

2. Understanding the Role of Genetic Testing

A small number of people have a much greater risk of developing aneurysms, and of having those aneurysms rupture, than the general population. If more people at high risk for aneurysms were identified through genetic studies, screening could be targeted to groups in which it is most likely to be beneficial. As medical experts, we are cautious about publicly available technologies. Generally speaking, we prefer that family members who are nervous about their risk of developing symptoms from non-genetic diseases not be genetically tested to give them reassurance that they are not at increased risk. Genetic testing should be conducted within a medical environment that helps those who may be affected by the knowledge that they carry a genetic mutation by providing the best possible prevention and treatment options.

Brain aneurysm usually does not cause any symptoms, so most aneurysms are discovered accidentally (for example, by imaging studies for unrelated problems). Some (but not all) aneurysms will rupture, causing a subarachnoid hemorrhage (SAH), which can carry up to a 50% chance of death. Aneurysms are frequently found in more than 5% of the population, but SAH occurs in only 10 of every 100,000 people in the United States and is most common in those ages 35 to 60. Although the relative risk of SAH during a lifetime is small, the public health burden of aneurysms and SAH is large because: Most people who have aneurysms are asymptomatic but are usually still at risk for developing a subsequent aneurysm. Many people feel anxious about their risk for aneurysms and the risk for SAH, especially if they have seen the consequences in a family member.

2.1. Principles of Genetic Testing

For the majority of brain aneurysm patients, whether or not their risk has a polygenic or a multifactorial genetic component (i.e., or both), having an affected relative is by far the best indicator of increased risk. Few genes have been identified with a monogenic substantially prevalent effect on aneurysm susceptibility; most first-degree relatives of a brain aneurysm patient have no identifiable mutations that would allow personalized risk information.

ADPKD has also been associated with CHD1L, but other CHDs have not been observed in such individuals. Genetic testing is not appropriate for everyone, however. One reason is that many factors are involved in aneurysm susceptibility that are not under any known genetic control. An example is the correlation with smoking. Another reason that genetic testing is not appropriate for everyone is that these genetic results indicate that the aneurysms that occur in association with the mutations are not necessarily identical to, or easily quantifiable together with, typical aneurysms, as they occur in an elevated predisposition monogenic population.

The molecular genetics of brain aneurysms are beginning to be elucidated via linkage studies, candidate gene studies, and rare mutation discovery efforts. While it is not currently possible to accurately quantify disease risk or make treatment decisions for any of the identified mutations, those individuals carrying a mutation are likely at significantly increased risk for brain aneurysms. In those individuals, earlier aneurysm screening might be beneficial.

2.2. Types of Genetic Tests Available for Brain Aneurysm Risk Assessment

Genetic testing can be offered for patients that have a family history of brain aneurysms. Aneurysm is when a blood vessel bulges weakly in the brain wall and can rupture, leading to stroke or death. Ruptured brain aneurysm has high rates of mortality, morbidity, and disability. The condition is not completely understood in regards to causes at this moment. In most cases, the aneurysm is asymptomatic and is usually discovered incidentally during other procedures. When a brain aneurysm is detected by MRA or CTA, surgical intervention is considered according to size and risk of the aneurysm. Having a family history leads to even more risk for the disease. The population with a family history of aneurysm has approximately 5% prevalence.

There are several types of genetic tests available. The type of genetic variations detected by a genetic test determines the clinical utility of a test. Genetic tests for assessing brain aneurysm risk are important when ordering a genetic test. Genetic testing for brain aneurysm risk is based on the detection of genetic variations known to be associated with the condition. Genetic variations associated with conditions are obtained by large population studies, and are usually identified using Genome-Wide Association Study (GWAS).

3. Indications for Genetic Testing in Individuals with Family History

Individuals who have family histories associated with an aneurysm are ideal candidates for preventive screening for unruptured aneurysm with invasive or noninvasive imaging tests after establishing a causal pathogenic variant in the family. The cost-effectiveness of such noninvasive imaging tests would encourage primary care providers to refer individuals with a family history for premortem genetic testing. However, the choice of any testing modalities cannot replace the original genetic testing goal to diagnose individuals with hereditary brain aneurysm at an early age and to allow prevention of deadly aneurysms. Thus, preferentially for individuals with a family history, above imaging-only screening for asymptomatic brain aneurysm.

Genetic testing for hereditary risk of brain aneurysm is recommended for individuals with a family history who meet the following clinical criteria: two or more relatives with a brain aneurysm or one case of brain aneurysm in an individual with a history of subarachnoid hemorrhage. Additionally, referral for genetic assessment is appropriate in cases of a solid family history of sudden death from an unknown cause, particularly if other family members have a known aneurysm phenotype. In the absence of a known pathogenic variant in the family, genetic testing may not be informative. Ruptured intracranial aneurysms are secular extraindividual variables that may reflect differences in underlying phenotypes or nonpolygenic risk factors for brain aneurysm rupture related to sex, age, tobacco use, or blood pressure.

3.1. Risk Factors and Red Flags for Brain Aneurysms

Individuals with a family history of brain aneurysms have an elevated risk of developing a brain aneurysm and should be alert for certain symptoms and tell a healthcare provider about them. Common symptoms of brain aneurysm include the sudden onset of an unusual headache, seizure, neck pain, or vision changes. These symptoms often require rapid medical attention. More informally, some people with a brain aneurysm experience a "violent" headache (sometimes called the "worst headache of my life headache") shortly before the brain aneurysm ruptures, but other people with a ruptured aneurysm do not recall having a particular headache beforehand.

A family history of a brain aneurysm is a significant risk factor for developing an aneurysm. The risk of an aneurysm in people with a family history is approximately 12%. This is 2% higher than the baseline risk of 10%, which is the probability of the general population developing a brain aneurysm over their lifetime. Genetic factors can contribute to the prevalence of brain aneurysms in some families by making the blood vessel walls of people more susceptible to defects such as weakening and bulging that trigger aneurysm formation. Researchers are still investigating the link between genes and these vascular problems. Brain aneurysm formation may be caused by a combination of genetic and environmental factors.

2) Differential diagnosis: A broad clinical spectrum, from highly penetrant disorders with a potentially detectable genetic cause (such as autosomal dominant polycystic kidney disease and Ehlers-Danlos syndrome), to individuals who simply represent phenocopies or carry only a portion of genetic susceptibility to intracranial aneurysm, has been reported. In addition, various causative and non-causative variants in various modifiable genes and background diseases attaching neural vessel dilatation have been implicated. The informed genetic counselor or therapist serves as a guide, linking neurovascular and cardiovascular specialists, genetic specialists, and other specialists such as radiologists and nephrologists. Prompt information on the differential diagnosis of conditions that are similar to each other is essential. The position statement by the Cerebrovascular Disorders Journal Association, The Japan Neurosurgical Society, and The Japanese Society for Neuroendovascular Therapy (JPNAT) in 2017, as well as the guidelines and consensus statements issued in Western countries, should be considered.

1) Gene(s) of interest: The timing and sensitivity of the genetic testing model may largely depend on which gene is being tested. Because MRA is a low-cost, noninvasive test that can be implemented at almost any point in time, deciding the gene(s) of interest and the ideal timing of detection for these genes is important in genetic testing for individuals with a family history. Risk-benefit analyses are

advised in settings where newborn screening is indicated to yield the opportunity for early treatment and reduced morbidity, relieve the psychological burden, and incentivize reproductive decision making.

4. The Genetic Counseling Process

There has been a case where two monozygotic twins harbored identical aneurysm-related pathogenic variants in the family. One of the twins chose genetic testing combined with pre-implantation genetic diagnosis following genetic counseling and prenatal genetic diagnosis in the next stage. A genetically healthy baby for pathogenic variants was conceived, and the family avoided repetition of the genetic risk of the aneurysm. The involvement of genetic counseling in the genetic diagnosis of hereditary aneurysm not only provides the necessary genetic medical service, educational supervision, disease risk, and disease management recommendations but also ensures that genetic information has been used in accordance with relevant medical ethics and laws, which are highly concerned by the public and the medical community today.

Genetic counseling is an essential and valuable part of genetic testing in familial aneurysm. Genetic counseling provides patients and families with accurate, innovative, and high-quality genetic medical services, health education to understand genetic diseases, disease-related information, evaluations, expressions, and management methods, and professional medical counseling to face the risk of disease. Genetic testing has extended the genetic services of health evaluation, medical disease consultation, disease risk assessment, treatment guidance, and family planning, and has a great impact on aspects from prenatal diagnosis to pre-implantation genetic diagnosis.

4.1. Importance of Genetic Counseling

The consequences of a positive genetic test for a known familial AN disease-causing mutation are different than they are for many other symptomatic diseases. This is in large part due to the limitations in predicting who will rupture and who will not in advance of the bleeding event. However, the clinical consequences of a positive test in a known familial mutation carrier are equally unique. Given this, all guidelines proposed by international societies who are knowledgeable about genetic testing for familial predisposition to symptomatic disease recommend that it is ideal, preferred, and in almost all cases essential to have pretest counseling. High on the list of reasons why this is the case include providing the family with an understanding of at-risk and not at-risk status, information about the meaning of a negative result, and the implications of either a negative or positive result. However, it is not necessary to stop the search for a disease-causing mutation in a family when it is taking too long to find or if a mutation is not located. All coding regions and intron-exon boundaries of nine genes can now be sequenced to identify disease-causing mutations using next-generation sequencing strategies. This offers new hope for increasing the diagnostic yield in some families with multiple affected members.

Genetic testing is an important step in identifying mutation carriers and providing accurate risk assessment, but it should not be done lightly. Confirmation of a mutation in any family must be done using appropriate clinical laboratory standards. The family must be apprised of the meaning and potential implications of a positive, equivocal, or uninformative negative result. It is important to remember that what may be a mutation in one family might, in fact, be a benign polymorphism if seen in another family. And while a risk factor can be established, the age of onset can be predicted, and long-term preventive measures exist, the most critical question – what will determine whether I or my family member will be one who ruptures an aneurysm and who will not? – cannot be answered with any assurance. Therefore, the decision to embark on familial testing and the resulting genetic testing should be part of a thoughtful, carefully considered process in consultation with a healthcare provider knowledgeable in the genetics of intracranial aneurysm.

4.2. Components of a Genetic Counseling Session

In a genetic counseling session before brain aneurysm genetic testing, genetic counselors work with you on education and counseling about different topics. Sometimes you need a conference, like a team conference. You work with the doctors of the genetics team, including a neurologist, a neurosurgeon, and/or an interventional neuroradiologist. In some meetings, a research nurse and/or a social worker may also be part of the team meeting. The information from the team meeting is put into letters. This information is of benefit to you and your healthcare providers. All the healthcare professionals are ready in advance to help you if you want genetic testing. You know who to go to in order to get the genetic testing. You also know what to do after you get the genetic testing. You can ask for a team exchange. There is someone to call. You know that the best interest of you and your family is the main goal of the team session.

It is a specialty in healthcare, like cardiology. It provides information about medical risks for the future, like genetic testing for health problems. It helps parents who have a child with a disability with difficulties of child care. You meet a genetic counselor for many hours, face to face. You can ask questions and get many answers. A genetic counselor has a degree in genetic counseling. The team has many people: genetic counselors, doctors, nurses, social workers, psychologists, research nurses, and others. Some genetic counselors work with researchers. They help the genetic research. They recruit, or ask, for people's help with genetic research. We need to find out why brain aneurysms happen. We need to help people have the best future possible.

5. Benefits and Limitations of Genetic Testing

The statistical chance for a mutation-positive individual to develop one or more IAs during his or her lifetime in a family known to have a particular familial mutation is much higher than the chance of the general population to develop an IA at some point in their life. Screening surveillance and possible other medical or surgical interventions to prevent rupture or re-rupture are then far more likely to be justified when the genetic test indicates the mutation is present. This justification arises, in part, from the fact that medial familial intracranial aneurysms commonly rupture at earlier ages than is typically observed for sporadic non-familial aneurysms. A ruptured brain aneurysm can cause a devastating stroke or, in patients lucky enough to survive, the severe disability associated with intracerebral or subarachnoid hemorrhage.

The benefits and limitations of direct mutation analysis in the setting of a family history of intracranial aneurysm (IA) with a known mutation are very different from the benefits and limitations of genetic association studies that assess risk in the general population if no family history is present. Once a mutation causing a specific inherited predisposition to IA has been discovered in a family with a known history, the primary purpose for testing in that family is specifically to determine whether or not an at-risk family member carries the mutation because the test is highly predictive of the risk. Confirming that a known gene mutation is present can be medically actionable in that it can provide timely warning to a family member, with potential need for clinical intervention to prevent or reduce the impact of a catastrophic brain aneurysm.

5.1. Potential Benefits of Genetic Testing

Even after the emergency treatment in the hospital, a partner or spouse may be required to retire or take a leave of absence from work. Sadly, it is not often a leave of absence but a retirement from the workforce to become the primary caregiver. This is necessary because of the cognitive and behavioral changes usually associated with an aneurysm, craniotomy, or the aneurysm-coil location. If your family members have had a brain aneurysm, talk with them about the potential benefits for themselves and their family members for preventing stroke through knowing their FIAA risks. Even though you do not know the hereditary component in a family history, you should consider genetic testing if you have an increased risk. If you are not yet in the group with a known family history, others will have knowledge that can ease your mind while you wait to find out.

This is a definite opportunity to save lives, suffering, and the lifelong consequences of brain aneurysm bleeding. Many people have the opportunity to avoid a serious problem through a simple test. This opportunity is largely wasted today. If your family members have had a brain aneurysm, talk with them about the potential benefits for themselves and their family members for preventing stroke through knowing their FIAA risks. Encouraging testing for something that you hope will not be found can make difficult dinner conversations. However, it can save lives, suffering, and the lifelong consequences of a brain aneurysm bleeding. The greatest emotional and financial expense of stroke and the greatest loss in quality of life is not the cost of the stroke itself but the long-term burden of disability caregiving.

5.2. Limitations and Ethical Considerations

For these reasons, developing the tools and resources to encourage at-risk individuals who express a potential interest in identifying themselves can blind a dangerous family history and help tailor medical and surgical intervention recommendations. It is currently not recommended to undergo genetic testing if there is only a family history of brain aneurysm. It is currently not recommended to undergo genetic testing unless the brain health provider has first recommended medication or surgical intervention if needed based upon the identification of a brain aneurysm. However, some ethical considerations include whether the sample should be included in a biobank or how many genes will be sequenced at once. Participants in the stakeholder workshop overwhelmingly supported the development of a stakeholder group to further discuss these issues.

Approximately 15% of cases of brain aneurysm occur in patients with a family history of brain aneurysm, defined as two or more affected first-degree relatives. Other factors that can increase risk include certain genetic or heritable conditions and individuals who exhibit multiple brain aneurysms. The majority of individuals identified with a brain aneurysm are older than 30, and the majority of these aneurysms are smaller than 3mm in final size. If there is no family history of brain aneurysm, it is currently thought safe to not screen a person or intervene with surgical clipping or coil embolization if the aneurysm is less than 7mm in size and asymptomatic. If an individual identifies themselves as high-risk due to family history, and the individual is above the age of 20, then the individual may choose to have a brain aneurysm prescreening to determine if there is an unruptured aneurysm present.

6. Case Studies and Real-Life Examples

Once within the same family, we received genetic testing results from a different commercial laboratory on three family members on the paternal side. This laboratory had tested them for mutations at 1 gene. None of these family members were found to have a mutation of the examined gene. Family members have their DNA tested in their quest for reason. When negative results are received, a new gene will emerge that has been linked to brain aneurysms. Then there is also a large group of families that have no genes linked to their IA families. Without knowing our gene blindness, healthy family members are falsely reassured when they incur a negative screen.

We discovered a family with a TGF-β receptor 2 (TGFBR2) mutation. In total, 17 carriers of this mutation have undergone clinical testing. All 17 had findings of moyamoya and/or brain aneurysm(s) on magnetic resonance angiography (MRA). This family is among the 10%–30% of brain aneurysm families that exhibit features of moyamoya syndrome as part of the phenotype. An evidence-based guide is being used to determine how to best manage and follow the carriers of this mutation during the different stages of their lives. The only presymptomatic therapy that exists for treating the vascular lesions in brain aneurysm relatives is revascularization of the brain arteries. We are currently only recommending therapy for those with symptomatic moyamoya.

The following case reports serve as examples of the use of genetic testing and the association with a higher incidence of IA development, IA rupture, and FIA with brain aneurysms. Brain aneurysm screening could be considered in family members identified as having IA risk by genetic testing. The decision to undergo screenings should be considered on an individual basis considering the blessings of knowing diagnosis early and the curse of knowledge if no brain aneurysms are discovered.

6.1. Case Study 1: Genetic Testing Impact on Treatment Decisions

The patient was one of the first 100 or so families recruited to the Familial Intracranial Aneurysm (FIA) Program at Indiana University and was found to have an inferred ACoA aneurysm predisposition gene on chromosome 1. Her gene(s) could only be verified when the single nucleotide polymorphism haplotype that co-segregated with disease in her family was found in a sufficient number of additional implicated families. It took several years before enough high-risk ACoA aneurysm families were recruited to confirm the frequent genetic predisposition of ACoA aneurysm families and for the exact FIA gene AT/CT haplotype and sub-haplotypes to become known. The LOC387715 rs 12737203 T risk allele was found in 50% to 100% of FIA families - depending on the type of ACoA clinical syndrome and the racial makeup of the nuclear family under study. The allelic risk effect was greatest in sporadic Central nervous system (CNS) aneurysm patients with highest spatial performance cognitive function scores, then healthy control individuals, then unruptured spatial cognitive families, then ruptured spatial cognitive FIA families.

In this case study, we highlight a patient who presented with an unruptured 7 mm anterior communicating artery aneurysm (ACoA). Her brother had a fatal SAH from an ACoA aneurysm at the same age as she was at presentation. Given he was her only affected relative, she had a heart-to-heart talk with the treating interventional neuroradiology doctor and decided to forego the recommended surgical therapy. She wondered why in this era of rapidly advancing medical technology he used the term "familial", as her highly trained neurologist brother was not in the habit of throwing out terminology without a strong basis for believing it was true. As the ethnicity and life insurance of family members would be impacted by her ACoA genetic risk status, she wanted to know whether the medical community could prove that her brother and three young sons had a much higher than the average population ACoA aneurysm risk.

6.2. Case Study 2: Family Screening and Risk Reduction Strategies

The patient was informed that there is no test that can predict brain rupture. The natural history of brain aneurysm is that about 1/3 of brain aneurysms will burst. Most importantly, having the anatomic lesion (brain aneurysm) as a reversible risk factor, it is imperative to use modern diagnostic tools, like with MRI/MRA, to image relatives at risk, and use associated strategies for brain aneurysm detection and management before aneurysm rupture occurs. Because most case patients are (fortunately) asymptomatic at the time of discovery, health care providers should take special care to "do no harm" and continually assess risk based on factors like calculable risk and life expectancy once risk reduction surgery is completed. Clearly, a first note on strategy is that this family has an illness with a diagnosis of exclusion, one which invokes occasional human errors with potentially very dire consequences. Family DRD is the most cost effective strategy to use for families with this represent diagnostics dilemma.

In this case, a 46-year-old woman has a family history of a brain aneurysm (Figure 1) and undergoes a genetic test (positive result) that is associated with a 50% risk for brain aneurysm. Of note, the phenotype is that of subarachnoid hemorrhage following rupture of an aneurysm and the identified genetic variant was a common polymorphism. What should be discussed when managing this individual?

7. Future Directions in Genetic Testing for Brain Aneurysm Risk

7.1. Emerging Technologies and Research Areas